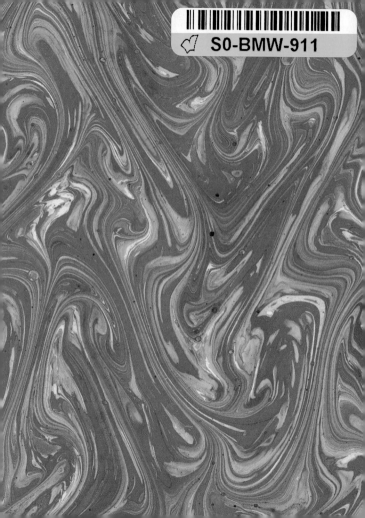

S0-BMW-911

A *COMPENDIUM* OF
ORIENTAL
HEALING

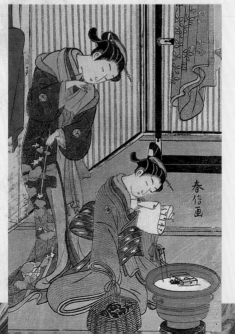

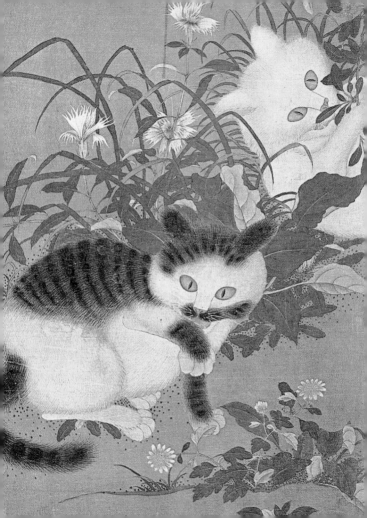

A GIFT OF *H*EALTH

A *COMPENDIUM* OF
ORIENTAL
HEALING

CHINESE HERBAL MEDICINE:
MANIPULATION & ACUPUNCTURE:
YOGA & MEDITATION, *ETC.*, *ETC.*

COMPILED AND
VISUALLY EMBELLISHED
FROM ORIGINAL SOURCES BY
W. CRAIG DODD ESQ.

NEW
HOLLAND

First published in 1996 by New Holland (Publishers) Ltd
London • Cape Town • Sydney • Singapore

24 Nutford Place, London W1H 6DQ, United Kingdom

80 McKenzie Street, Cape Town 8001, South Africa

3/2 Aquatic Drive, Frenchs Forest, NSW 2086, Australia

Distributed by Sterling Publishing Company, Inc
387 Park Avenue South, New York, NY 10016

Distributed in Canada by Sterling Publishing
c/o Canadian Manda Group, One Atlantic Avenue, Suite 105,
Toronto, Ontario, Canada M6K 3E7

ISBN 1 85368 669 7

Editor: Michele Brown
Designer: Craig Dodd
Editorial Direction: Yvonne McFarlane

Reproduction by Hirt and Carter, Cape Town, South Africa
Printed and bound in Singapore by Tien Wah Press Ptd Ltd

This is not a medical book. It is a gift book. It is not intended to
replace the services of a physician, nor is it meant to encourage diagnosis
and treatment of illness, disease or other medical problems by the layman.
Any application of the recommendations set out in the following pages is at
the reader's discretion and sole risk. If under a physician's care, they will
advise if any recommendations are suitable for you. Pregnant women are
advised to avoid all drugs - synthetic or herbal.

CONTENTS

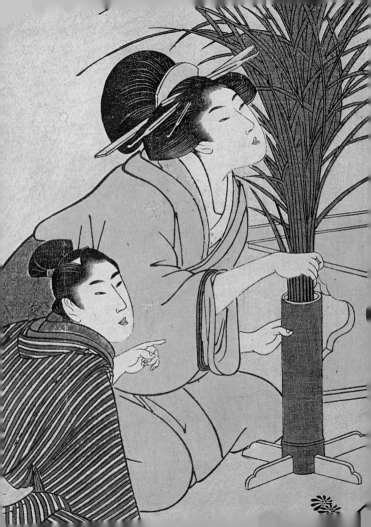

PREFACE

Within the pages of the Small Volumes which comprise **A Gift of Health,** there is contained the Collected Wisdom of Sages and Savants, Herbalists and Sensualists from throughout the Ages.

From their very Words the Modern Reader may glean much **Useful Information** to help with the **Problems of Everyday Life**, be they Physical or Psychological.

This very volume offers a Tantalizing Insight into a Particular World of **Life Enhancing Wisdom** as do the Companion Volumes.

A Garden of Herbal Remedies takes you along the Pathways of the Healing Herbal Garden. The Wisdom of the Ancient Herbalists being distilled to illuminate this Healing Art. The Potency of Each and Every Herb herein is defined, together with a Veritable Pharmacopocia of Nature's Remedies to lead to a Healthier Life.

A Compendium of Oriental Healing takes you into the Erudite World of the Ancient Healing Arts of the Orient. The Mysteries of Acupuncture, Meditation, Moxibustion and the Oldest of Herbal Cures are explained, together with the Ways of Ayurvedic Medicine which treats the Whole Person rather than an Isolated Disease.

A Bouquet of Aromatherapy is a Celebration of the Healing, Soothing and Sensual Qualities of the Plant Kingdom. It offers a Perfumed Voyage through the World of Essential Oils, their Uses, Practical applications and Healing Properties. It also features Dr. Bach's Flower Remedies and, on a lighter note, the Creation of Personal Pot-pourri and Fragrances.

A Cornucopia of Aphrodisiacs combines many of the Features of the aforesaid Companion Volumes, bringing together Folklore and Fancy, Enchanting Elixirs and Arousing Recipes to Enhance the Libido and Promote a Joyful Union of Partners.

Taken together, ingested and digested, the Messages from Across the Aeons of Time will truly prove to be **A Gift of Health**.

W. Craig Dodd

The Author thanks Michael Mitchell Johnstone of that Ilk for his Painstaking Research without which this Estimable Volume would have remained Unwritten.

LEGACY OF THE YELLOW EMPEROR

For two millenia **Chinese Medicine** has been recorded and refined for the treatment of the **Mind** as much as the **Body**. The first **Major Treatise** to codify remedies is the *Huang Ti Nei Ching* or the *Yellow Emperor's Canon of Internal Medicine*. **Huang Ti**, the Eponymous Yellow Emperor, was the third of three legendary emperors associated with Chinese medicine.

The first, **Fu Hsi**, is credited with the formulation of the **Yin** and the **Yang**, the cornerstone of **Chinese Philosophy**. The second, **Shen Nung** is said to have invented the plough and penned a herbal entitled *Shen Nung Pen Ts'ao*, based on his own experimentation. Popular Legend has it that this Most Worthy of Men meandered through field, marsh and forest every day conducting his researches on Native Botanicals, poisoning himself up to eighty times a day and using his Legendary Physic Powers to cure himself.

Huang Ti is said to have invented the first wheeled vehicle, ships, a planetarium, cloth, clothing, and musical notation, as well as finding time to write his Highly Regarded Treatise. The receipts contained therein pre-date similar concoctions of Western Alchemists by almost one thousand years.

A Millenium after the Sad Demise of Huang Ti, I-Yin, a cook in the imperial kitchens, served a decoction of several different herbs to the court. It was Much Appreciated, not only for its flavour, but also for its beneficial side effects. Such decoctions soon became the most popular way of administering drugs, establishing I-Yin as the originator of the Herb Teas and Soups (T'ang) that are of Such Importance in Oriental Medicine.

Although everyday ailments were treated, the Alchemists had in common an Ultimate Goal – to find the Elixir of Immortality. In their Pursuit of what we now know to be an Unattainable Quest they flirted with death, deformity and danger as they were prepared to use any potion which might result in the Magical Crystalline Pill. Several Chinese Emperors, as well as the Alchemists themselves, succumbed to fatal doses of mystical potions, so great was their desire for immortality. One of the greatest killers was Mercury and Compounds thereof. The frequency with which this Liquid Metal was used as the Principal Ingredient of many a concoction suggests that the Alchemists did not consider it dangerous at all when mixed with various other Exotic, but Harmless, ingredients.

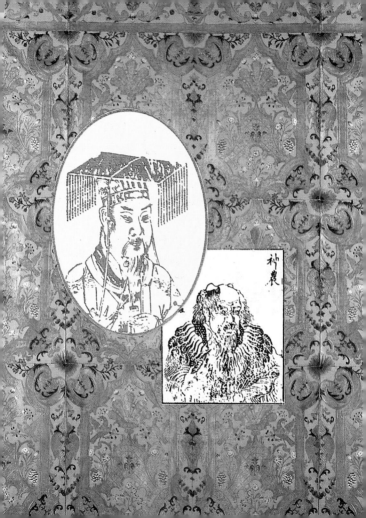

神農

In the Tan Ching Yao Chuch, *The Book of Essential Formulas*, of the 7th century, Alchemists were directed to 'take jujube paste, powdered rhinoceros horn, musk, cinnabar and sulphur and mix with mercury . . . to be rolled into pillules the size of hempseeds.' This potentially deadly concoction was supposed to cure every condition from Anxiety to Attacks of the Heart, from Dropsy to Demonic Possession.

Precious Metals and various others were powdered and Incorporated into the Elixirs, the more precious, the more efficaceous they were thought to be. The more spiritually inclined Alchemists saw these metals as only external symbols of deeper reality, for the Great Essential of all Chinese Medicine is the balancing of the universal opposites Yin and Yang, a deeper understanding of which is essential to Full Knowledge of the Healing Arts of the Orient.

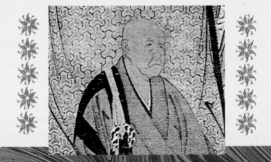

AFORE YIN AND YANG

The Ultimate Concept of Chinese Medicine has no Equal in **Occidental Medicine**. It is the concept of **Qi**, represented in Chinese Literature as a **Serpentine Symbol**. The **Power of Qi** is Totally Pervasive. It is the Essential Life-Force of Mankind and Encompasses all the Vital Activities, Spiritual, Emotional, Mental and Physical. It keeps the Blood and Bodily fluids flowing; it warms the body; it fights disease. Qi force flows along channels within the body forming a continuous circuit linking all parts of the body. It is to these channels that the skilled *Acupuncturist* will apply his trusted needles.

Qi has two complementary aspects much more widely known, but often not fully understood by those in the Occident – the **Yin** and the **Yang**.

According to the Esteemed Yellow Emperor's *Canon of Internal Medicine*, 'Yin Yang is the basic principle of the entire universe. It is the principle of everything in creation. It brings about all change: it is the root source of Life and Death, it is found within the **Temples of the Gods**. Through their Interactions and Functions, Yin and Yang, the negative and positive principle in nature, are responsible for the diseases which befall those who are in rebellion against the laws of nature.'

Yin and Yang are relative terms and all Phenomena have a Yin and Yang Aspect. There can be no Yin without Yang, just as there is no Night without Day. The Classic Chinese hieroglyphic character for Yang shows the Sun with shining rays and a mountain. A mountain is represented in the character for Yin, but it is combined with a cloud.

The healthy body is in constant change from Yin to Yang and from Yang to Yin. Nothing is Neutral: either Yin or Yang is in excess, but if the excess goes unchecked, disease arises. Illnesses due to excessive Cold penetrating the body, pallor, chilled extremities are Yin Conditions. Those with signs of heat, flushes and fevers, are Yang. The Prescribed Treatment will aim to re-establish a balance of Yin and Yang.

Those who have studied the **Pharmacopoeia** of the **East** have access to a Richness of Herbal Remedies to cure anything with which the body may be stricken. And as each herb has its own Yin Yang properties, combining them gives Myriad Miraculous Cures.

According to Yin Yang, each disease follows the same cycle which, if it goes unchecked, may lead to death. At the first stage, the Big Yang Stage, **Tai Yang**, the disease

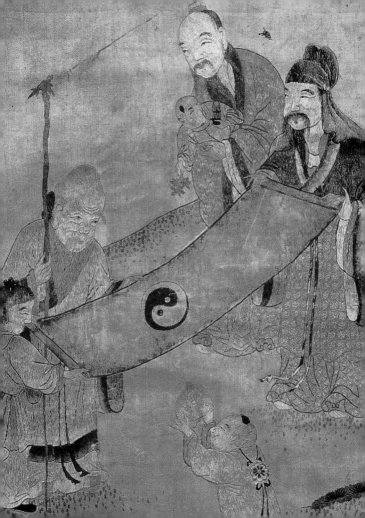

has not penetrated the body's defences: it is in the skin and muscles. At the second stage, the Small Yang, **Shao Yang**, the disease is half inside the body, half outside, and by the third stage, the Clear Yang, **Yang Ming**, it may have entered the Meridians of the Stomach and Intestines. By the Big Yin, **Tai Yin**, stage, the spleen will have been affected to the Detriment of the Workings of the Stomach. In the Small Yin, **Shao Yin**, stage, the disease has entered the heart and kidneys and by the Receding Yin Stage, **Chueh Yin**, all the organs are affected especially the liver. Death may soon follow.

Yin has Connotations of Softness, Darkness, Coldness and Wetness.

Yang has connotations of Hardness, Brightness, Heat and Dryness.

If you are healthy, Yin and Yang are in a State of Flux, constantly balancing each other.
Daily Activity is a Yang State.
Sleeping is a Yin state.

MAGIC NEEDLES

ă'cŭpŭncture *n.* (Med.) (orig. Chinese) method of pricking skin or tissues with needles as treatment for various conditions. [f. L *acu* with a needle + PUNCTURE]

According to Legends of the Orient, over 4,500 years before the word **Acupuncture** became substantive in the English Language, many Chinese Warriors who survived the misfortune of being struck by arrows whilst in battle recorded that while they were sorely injured, troublesome agues, aches and pains in other parts of the body which had afflicted them previously lessened in intensity and even were miraculously cured.

Similarly, **Tribesmen** of the **African Plains** had long been exhorted by their *Shaman*, or **Witchdoctor**, to treat an ailment of one part of the body by piercing another part of their anatomy, seemingly unrelated to their particular complaint. In the **Frozen Wastes** of the **Arctic** and the **Northern Tundra** worthy anthropologists concerned with the welfare of the **Inuit Peoples** have reported the use of sharp stones put to similar use: the earliest Chinese 'needles', similarly, were in fact shards of stone. In the **Tropical Rainforests** of **Amazonia** one tribe has, since the Dawn of

Time, used **Blowpipes** to insert Tiny Arrows into one part of the body to cure a malady in another; many of the points coinciding with those used by the Chinese.

The literature pertaining to the subect is as extensive as the subject is old. The earliest known text on this most ancient of medical skills is the *Nei Ching*, a scroll reputed to be the work of Hunga Ti, the aforementioned Yellow Emperor. Using the medical knowledge he so assiduously garnered he lived into his ninth decade, ascending to the Heavens in 2596 BC.

We know from this and other writings that acupuncturists of old used nine needles:

* the Arrowhead needle, for superficial pricking
* the Round needle, for massaging
* the Blunt needle for pressing
* the Sharp Three-Edged needle for pricking veins
* the Sword-like needle for releasing pus
* the Sharp and Round needle for rapid pricking
* the Filiform needle for general use
* the Long needle for puncturing thick muscle
* the Large needle for treating arthritis

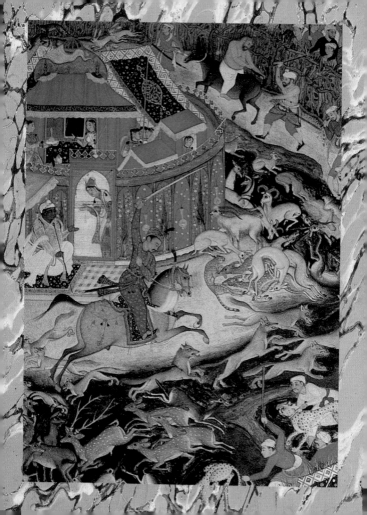

Several of these needles have long fallen Into Disuse or have been refined from their earlier shape, but a set discovered in 1968 in the tomb of the Much Lamented Liu Sheng, dating from the 200BC, shows that some of the implements used by Acupuncturists are the same now as they were then.

The underlying principle of Acupuncture is that all diseases cause a corresponding part of the body, an acupuncture point, to become inflamed; the inflammation disappears when the disease is cured.

As with all things Chinese, the Yin, Yang and Qi lie at the very Heart of the Matter. Qi energy, the Very Essence of the life force, flows through channels in the body called **Meridians** which may overlap with, but are quite distinct from, the central Nervous and Circulatory Systems. The energy courses around the body in a well-defined circle from meridian to meridian and from organ to organ.

The amount of Qi flowing through the meridians varies from time to time as do the Ratios of Yin and Yang. When Imbalances Occur, the result is illness. The acupuncturist uses the needles to restore harmony to the system thus Effecting a Cure.

Those who look to Acupuncture in their Quest for Cures believe not only that each part of the body has both Yin and Yang qualities, but also that each of the five major of Ts'ang organs, the liver, the heart, the spleen, the lungs and the kidneys, are associated with its own element, respectively wood, fire, earth, metal and water. There are, in addition, two further organs to which are ascribed Mystical and Metaphysical properties – **The Triple Warmer** and **The Gate of Life**.

The Triple Warmer is a Yin Organ, sometimes called 'The Burning Spaces' and is believed to regulate the organs and the flow of Vital Fluids. Its properties are balanced by the Yang of the Grace of Life which is linked to happiness and joy and is the root of the Sexual Impulse.

When they considered the main Meridians of the Qi, the early acupuncturists divided the body into six major divisions, three Yang and three Yin, each of which encompassed two Major Meridians.

These Main Meridians are connected by fifteen 'Luo' Channels, and in addition there are other meridians numbering perhaps 47, including one that runs down the front of the body and another extending from the base of the skull to the coccyx. The number of acupuncture points on each meridian varies, and although they all affect the particular organ, it is not necessarily in the same manner.

Early texts refer to 365 acupuncture points and as the science, for surely that is what it is, developed, more points were discovered and that number has increased Almost Threefold.

In acupuncture, consultation, examination and diagnosis are of Equal Importance to the actual treatment. The physician begins the consultation by talking to the patient, focussing on the History of the Problem, the Symptoms, the patient's general physical, mental and emotional health.

When the consultation has come to a conclusion, the acupuncturist takes the patient's pulse three times at each wrist. In so doing, much knowledge about the disposition of Qi and imbalances of Yin and Yang is garnered.

After the pulses have been taken, the physician examines the patient's tongue, the appearance of which, and any coatings thereon, providing skilled practitioners with valuable information about the location, strength and nature of any disease.

The diagnosis made, the acupuncturist knows into which acupuncture points his needles should be inserted. Most usually these points are located on the forearms, hands, lower legs and feet, although there are points on all parts of the body.

The needles are inserted and rotated gently, though some acupuncturists prefer to leave them stationary. The needles remain in such position for the required time, which may be a few seconds or several minutes.

Silver and Gold needles were the tools of the ancients; today most acupunturists use more Antiseptic Modern Materials. The needles, which must by law be sterilized before use, are inserted to a depth of around $\frac{1}{4}$in (6mm) depending on the patient's build, the part of the body concerned and whether the disorder being treated affects the exterior or interior of the body.

Using the Thorough Knowledge of Anatomy, the acupuncturist takes care to avoid needle contact with blood vessels or any of the body's major organs.

The Venerable Art of Acupuncture is practised by over half a million doctors in China where it is an integral part of that country's medical system. Major operations are carried out with the patient fully conscious, the part of the body being operated on having been completely numbed by the application of needles in relevant acupuncture points. It is also widely used by women to relieve the Pains of Labour.

Caveat the First
Those looking to acupuncture to cure their various maladies must tell those they consult if they are receiving orthodox drug treatment for their ills, for this makes tongue and pulse diagnosis unreliable.

Caveat the Second
Chinese skilled in the ways of acupuncture often combine their skills with the needles with their knowledge of herbal medicine. It is best to refrain from seeking acupuncture treatment while simultaneously submitting to other treatments – especially if it be for the same ailment.

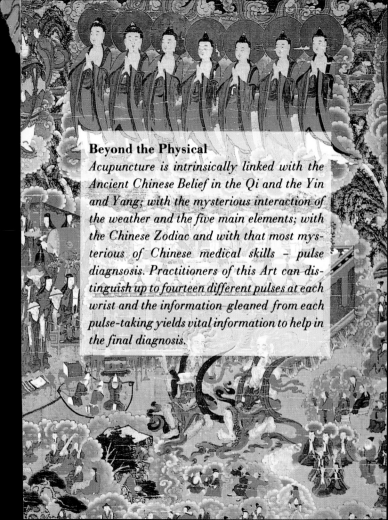

Beyond the Physical

Acupuncture is intrinsically linked with the Ancient Chinese Belief in the Qi and the Yin and Yang; with the mysterious interaction of the weather and the five main elements; with the Chinese Zodiac and with that most mysterious of Chinese medical skills – pulse diagnsosis. Practitioners of this Art can distinguish up to fourteen different pulses at each wrist and the information gleaned from each pulse-taking yields vital information to help in the final diagnosis.

MICROPUNCTURE

Those familiar with medical practices of times gone by may be aware that the practice of blood letting by the application of leeches was once widespread. The Chinese refrained from such a practice; they preferred the gentler practice of **micropuncture**, whereby a minute quantity of blood is removed from an appropriate acupuncture point, often with instant and amazing effect. Those of a sceptical nature may scoff, but anyone whose overenthusiastic devotions at the Temple of Bacchus have resulted in a heavy head and who submit themselves to having but one drop of blood withdrawn from the finger terminal of the large intestine meridian will testify to the efficacy of micropuncture.

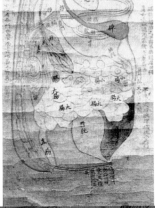
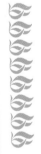

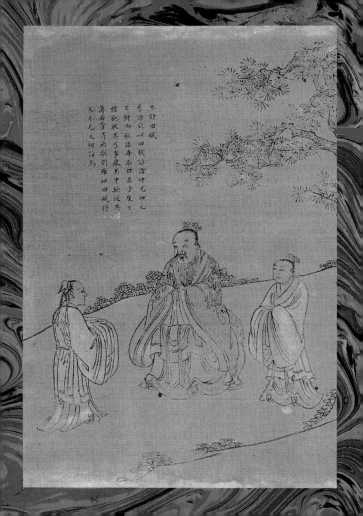

MOXIBUSTION

This most economical and practical treatment warms and tonifies the body's Qi and is particularly efficacious in cool, humid climates where the body's energy circulates at a deeper level than in warmer, drier climes. Hence its popularity in Japan, where it is widely used for home treatments.

Traditionally, a cone of **moxa**, the dried leaves of common mugwort, is placed on the chosen spot and ignited with the burning end of an incense stick. The heat penetrates the acupuncture point and tonifies the Qi of the relevant meridian.

Moxas may be as large as a cherry or as small as a large grain of sugar. Large moxas are used to stimulate energy and are removed when the patient signals that the heat has become uncomfortable, before being reapplied, often several times in one session. Small moxas burn right down to the skin, causing a tiny blister that maintains the heat, thus making the stimulus last longer.

While the Japanese favour the use of small boxes, the Chinese prefer the use of the moxa stick, the glowing end of which is held close to the treatment point for as long as the patient can bear the burning sensation.

The Chinese also apply moxa through acupuncture needles. After the needles have been inserted, little balls of moxa are wrapped round the tip and ignited, thus warming the needles which conduct the Beneficial Heat through the meridian. Moxibustion Acupuncture produces a most pleasing sensation and is especially effective in bringing about pain relief, especially pain of the muscular type.

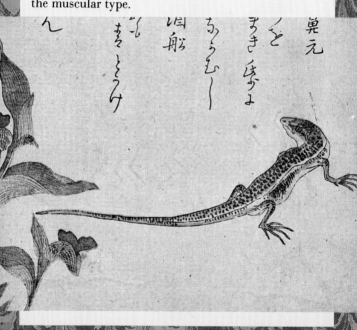

CUPPING

The Orient has long made use of a **Most Effective Method** of ridding the body of boils and abscesses, treating painful rheumatism and arthritis, banishing colds and chills, and helping those whose lungs are sore afflicted by asthma.

The process is known as **Cupping** and involves applying dome-shaped suction cups of different sizes to the body. Before their Actual Application, the Practitioner causes a piece of cotton material drenched in alcoholic spirit to catch fire, and uses forceps to hold the flaming torch at the mouth of the cup. The heat expands the air held inside the cup, some of which escapes, so that when it is positioned on the prescribed part and the air cools, a Partial Vacuum is created. This draws the flesh into the cup, causing an increased flow of blood and a resultant reddening of the skin. When the cups have been in position for the correct length of time, pressure is exerted on the skin around the cup, causing its release. Those who believe in the Yin and the Yang know that ridding the body of unwanted **Qi** Causes the Cure.

The cups were originally made of bamboo, but that Dragon, Scientific Technology, has made possible glass 'cups' the use of which is now widespread.

CHINESE HEALING HERBS

The legendary **Pharmacopoeia** of the **Chinese Herbal** spills over with abundant treatment for conditions ranging from Alopecia to Eczema: tonics for those for whom the Orgasm is unachievable and for those who, in their sexual enthusiasm, are unable to gain mastery over its quicksilver surges: and Cures for those whose overindulgence at the Altar of Bacchus has caused their heads to ache. There is nothing that western medicine can offer that cannot be matched, or often improved, by consultation with one skilled in the **Alchemy** of **Chinese Herbal Medicine**.

Chinese Herbal Preparations are the great balancers of the body, keeping the **Yin** and the **Yang** in Harmony, ensuring that we optimise the Energies and Cosmic forces that course through our bodies. Rather than guaranteeing health and longevity, they promote them by improving the tone of the muscles, organs and body tissues: they stimulate the natural functions, encouraging the body as it ages to continue to enjoy the benefits of Food, Sexual Activity and Exercise.

The Prescriptions are usually applied in one of three methods – pill, powder or soup – *Wan, San* and *T'ang*.

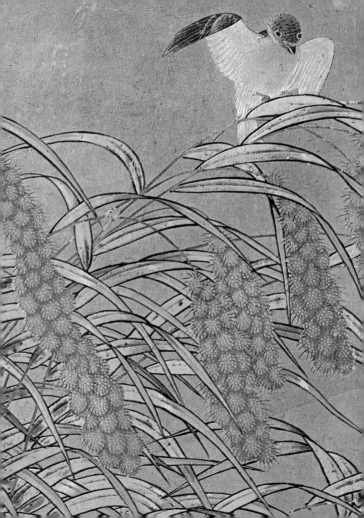

A Cornucopia of Cures

From humble reed grass and ordinary olive to glorious gardenia and legendary lotus, from venomous viper and dangerous dragon to scuttling scorpion and testudinal tortoise, many and varied are the flora and fauna used by the **Masters** of the **Chinese Herbal** in the preparation of their concoctions.

Let us pause for a moment to look in a Little Detail at the herbal cures that '**Calm the Liver and Stop the Wind**', from crushed Sea Shell to Broth of Scorpion, so wide is the range of remedies on the herbalist's shelves to calm the ascending liver yang and all the nervous systems attendant upon it.

To Calm the Liver is to bring its yin and yang into equilibrium. To stop the wind is to impede the nervous energy emanating from a troublous liver.

To this most vital of organs are ascribed the element Wood and the planet Jupiter; the colour Green and the taste Sour; the climate of Wind and the eastern direction; a rancid Odour and an angry Emotion; the barnyard Fowl and the number Eight; Plum is its fruit and Shout its sound; its grain is Wheat.

Western physicians faced with a patient displaying fuzzy vision with black spots, blemished nails and muscular spasms would look to the liver to find the root cause. In Chinese eyes, sight, muscles and nails all belong to the element wood and reflect liver functions. But further, wood is associated with anger and depression, emotions to which those with overactive livers are prone, and which may cause them to raise the voice – shouting being the sound ascribed to wood.

A patient showing symptoms of ascending liver-yang along with giddiness, blurred vision, headache: convulsions and spasms; fever and delirium: and swollen painful eyes, should be prescribed horn of antelope.

If the liver-yang ascendency is accompanied only by dizziness, giddiness, blurred vision and hurtful, painful eyes it should be treated with powdered sea-ear shell of the *Haliotade* family.

Giddiness and fainting due to liver-yang ascendancy accompanied by convulsions, headaches and numbness will find relief in the rhizomes of *Gastrodia elata*. Women with child who are similarly afflicted should look to the stems and spines of *Uncaria rhynchophylla* for relief.

Attacks of hiccups, burping, vomitous nausea tinnitus, dizziness and headaches caused by ascending liver-yang should be less frequent after treatment by tinctures containing humble hematite.

Nostrums containing extract of earthworm act on the liver to cure nervous convulsions, wind pains, stroke paralysis, abdominal swelling and difficulties with urination.

A powder made from the deadly scorpion acts to sedate the liver when treating spasms and nervous convulsions, tetanus, abscesses and boils. The liver will also be sedated by either a powder or a broth made from the humble centipede.

Release Externally

Another major group of remedies are those that induce or increase perspiration to release 'evil-qui'. They are **Diaphoretic** in **Nature** and are used to dispel 'wind heat' or 'wind cold' symptoms.

The seventeen plants used so to do range from the Cinnamon Tree to the White Mulberry, from the Chysanthemum to the Black Soybean. The sole representation from the Animal Kingdom is the humble Cicada,which is used to treat cataracts and convulsions.

Afflictions that react beneficially to Diaphoretic Dosage include chills and fever, bronchial asthma and hay fever, diarrhoea and menstrual disorders, amongst others too numerous to mention in a Volume of This Nature.

The Beefsteak Plant is to be recommended to those suffering Allergic Reaction to Shellfish, while anyone Unfortunate enough to be bitten by a snake, should avail themselves of the roots of *Angelica Anomala*.

Relief of a Natural Nature

Those whose lives are made miserable by an inability to pass stool on a regular basis, if at all, may look to the Chinese Herbal for relief. The natural world offers an assortment of allies that encourage the elimination of stagnant food and unpassed faeces from the nether parts of the Digestive System. Such remedies are made from the rhizome of rhubarb and leaflet of Tinnevelly Senna, crystal of Glauber's Salt, and juice extracted from the leaves of the Curacao Aloe, from the seeds of hemp and kernels of the noble Chinese Plum tree's seeds, from the roots of *Euphorbia Kansui* and the seeds of both Blue Morning Glory and Purging Croton.

And Yet More

The other major groups of Remarkable Remedies are either antipyretic, aromatically dehydratory, diuretic, antirheumatic, cold dispelling, reviving, sedative, energy regulatory, blood regulatory, stomachic, digestive, expectoratory, anthelmintic or tonic in nature.

A Pair of Prescriptions

The efficacy of Chinese Herbal Medicines is Evidenced by the two prescriptions detailed below, the first for those whose puberty is blighted by unsightly acne; the second for whom the stresses and strains of twentieth-century life has caused their blood pressure to rise to Too High a level.

Both make sufficient liquid for one day's dosage.

Chinese persons of teenage years, desirous of banishing the pimples and pock marks of youth may ask their herbalist to prepare a lotion made by boiling ½oz (10gr) each of the appropriate part of *Angelica anomala* (root), *Angelica sinensis* (root), Baical Skullcap (root), Balloon Flower (root), Chinese Licorice (root), Chinese White Peony (root), Gardenia (mature fruit), Hare's Ear (root), Japanese Catnip (stems and leaves), *Ledebouriella seseloides* (root), *Ligusticum wallichii* (root), Trifoliate

Orange (unripe fruit) and Weeping Golden Bell (fruit) in five cups of water in a covered earthenware or ceramic pot over a low flame until it has decocted to three cups of liquid which is then strained and taken as prescribed.

Simpler is the receipt for the treatment of high blood pressure. 1½oz (30gr) each of Japanese Honeysuckle and Chrysanthemum flowers should be boiled in five cups of water in a covered pot along with 1oz (20gr) each of Tiger Thistles and Hawthorn fruits and ½oz (10gr) of White Mulberry leaves until it decocts to three cups. The strained liquid is taken twice a day on an empty stomach.

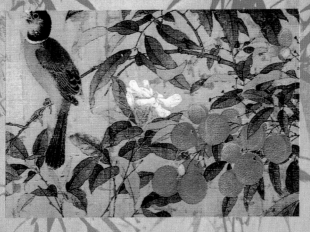

GINSENG

The List of Ailments said to benefit by taking this most noble of plants, *Panax Ginseng*, is as long as it is wide – from headaches to tiredness, amnesia to diabetes. It slows the ageing process, is a boon to those whose circulation is a problem and is said to encourage an increase in Sexual Desire.

Many and various, too, are the ways in which this Miraculous Root may be taken. In its root form it may be chewed: it may be administered as a pill or a powder, capsule or tablet or taken as a tea.

The plant, related to the humble ivy and American spikeyard, is much Cultivated in China, Korea and the eastern part of what was the once-mighty Russian empire. It prospers in damp, cool, humus-rich soil which encourages the Noble Root to grow to the desired length before it is Most Lovingly dug up and washed, after the outer tendrils have been removed.

Part of the crop will be steamed in an ages-old and Still Secret Process that reddens the root lending it a translucency of a most Attractive nature. The re-mainder, white ginseng, which retains its Yellow Hue and Opaque Nature, is slowly dried over many weeks.

Those who have partaken of Ginseng in one of its many forms sing its praises Most Highly. Those who may be considering its use should beware: plants from other parts of the world look to usurp its crown as king of medicinal plants. Two impostors from the New World, *Panax quinquefolium* and *pfaffia* (Brazilian ginseng) have their adherents, as does another from Russia, *Eleutherococcus senticosus* (Siberian ginseng). In truth, this Scurrilous Trio have some medicinal benefit, but those who have partaken of True Ginseng will hold with no other. Floreat *Panax ginseng*.

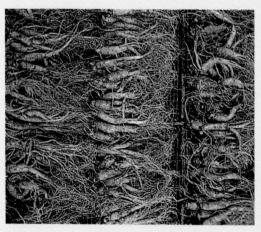

IN THE KITCHEN

To **Emily Post**'s remark that woman accepted cooking as a chore but man has made it a recreation, may be added 'and the Chinese made it a way of life.' For **Chinese Cuisine** is so closely associated with **Chinese Herbal Medicine** that the two are virtually inseparable. When the two are wed and consummate their nuptials in the kitchen, their offspring is an array of dishes that satisfy the needs of the belly and the dictates of health alike.

An example of this duality of purpose is **Ginseng Steamed Chicken Legs**, a dish that acts as a tonic, stimulant and aphrodisiac, promoting hormonal secretions and retarding ageing.

Halve three large chicken legs at the joint and cut each piece into two. Put in a heatproof dish and drench it in a cupful of rice wine or dry sherry. Add five slices of ginger and ½oz (10gr) of panax ginseng, place the bowl into a steam basket or steamer wok and steam over a high heat until an hour has passed. Meanwhile, mince two spring onions into individual soup bowls along with white pepper. When the meat is cooked, ladle it into these bowls along with the ginseng pulp and broth.

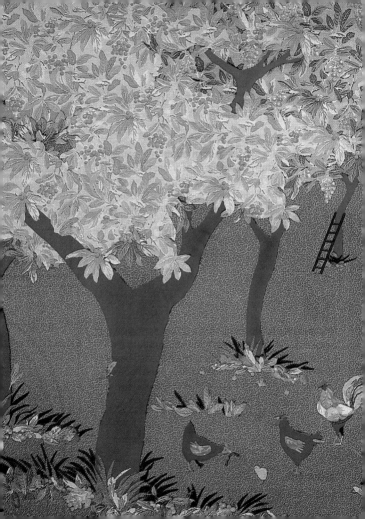

HEALING POWER OF HONEY IN HISTORY

The **Ancient Egyptians** widely used **Honey** as a **Medicinal Aid**. A Papyrus of *Various Medical Lore* dating back some 3500 years lists near on one thousand remedies. In more than half of them Honey is an Important Ingredient, particularly valued in salves mixed with vegetable oils or animal fats.

To the Chagrin of some Modern Sceptics, recent experiments have shown that the Ancient Egyptian Apothecaries were correct to place so much faith in it, a faith which has been handed down in folk medicine over the centuries. It can soothe a wound and speed healing. It readily absorbs water, thus drying a wound and promoting the Growth of Healthy Tissue. Since it is a Potent Killer of Harmful Bacteria, honey defies decay and has been found still Moist and Golden in Urns and Pots of tombs as old as two thousand years. The honey had been preserved by its own Purity.

It takes the nectar of some one and a half million blossoms to produce one pound of this viscous liquid, known in the East as *The Food of the Gods*, the use of which was advocated by King Solomon, *viz*: 'Eat thou honey which is good, and the honeycomb which is sweet.'

It has long been used in the treatment of burns and other skin problems and is a valuable ally in the restoration of health by those suffering from problems arising from the kidneys, from poor circulation of the blood or from anaemia.

Chinese sages, well-versed in medical knowledge, have long regarded honey as a yin-tonic and advocated the taking of their cures in the form of honey pills. After the necessary herbs have been ground into powder and the honey boiled and skimmed, the two are mixed into a smooth dough. This is then rolled into long, thin tubes, a small part of which is pinched off and rolled between finger and thumb into the traditionally shaped pills.

Honey has also long been used as an aid to beauty. Women of the Occident desirous of adding softness to the skin and lustre to the complexion can do little better than look to their Oriental Sisters who, for centuries, have spread it over their faces and waited for a quarter of one hour before gently removing with sponge and water.

A BESTIARY OF BENEFITS

Eye of newt and toe of frog,
Wool of bat and tongue of dog.
Adder's fork and blind-worm's sting.
Lizard's leg and howlet's wing

Those familiar with the **Scottish Play** could be forgiven for assuming that the crones who prophesied the rise of the Thane of Glamis to be the King of Scotland, and his subsequent downfall, were familiar with the **Chinese Herbal**. Had the play been the work of a Chinese Bard, the witches' incantation could well have read:

Horn of rhino, scale of pangolin,
Corpse of snake, gizzard of hen.
Shell of tortoise, eggcase of mantis,
Antler of deer, hide of ass.

for it is not only the flora of the Orient that composes the Chinese Herbal: the fauna plays its part, too . . .

Antelope (ling yang jiao) The powdered horn is used in the treatment of liver complaints: it reduces fever, sharpens the eyesight and soothes spasms. Pills containing the powder may be prescribed in the treatment of high blood pressure and are effective in the prevention of strokes.

Ass (e jiao) The glue prepared from the hide of *Equus Asinus* tones the blood and soothes painful lungs.

Centipede (wu gong) Many experts opine that the humble centipede is an excellent ally in the battle against various cancers. It is also an antispasmodic and antidote to snake bites. Women expectant of child should avoid any contact with concoctions made from the centipede.

Chicken (ji nei jun) The gastric tissue of the gizzard improves digestive functions by tonifying the stomach and distributing beneficial nutrients around the body. When dry, fried with lumps of charcoal, it eases the pain caused by mouth abscesses.

Cicada (chan tui) A powder made from the molten carapace of this insect, when dissolved in water is efficacious in the treatment of fever and spasms. Mixed with *Chrysanthemum morifolium*, the same powder helps those whose sight is dulled by cataracts.

Dragon bones (long gu) With nomenculture from Ancient Times, any fossilized bone, when crushed to a powder, is a useful astringent and sedative. Applied externally the powder has an effective styptic action on sores and abscesses.

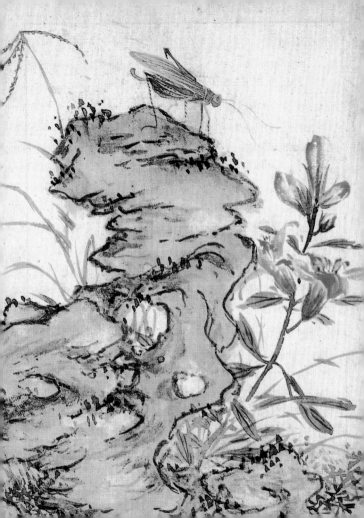

Earthworm (qui yin) A solution based on the common earthworm sedates the liver, clears the bronchial passages, reduces fever and increases the flow of urine. It also reduces high blood pressure by softening hardened veins and arteries.

Musk (she xiang) A dried secretion of the preputial follicles of the musk deer helps maintain a healthy heart and good circulation and is a welcome stimulant for those overburdened by the cares of the world.

Pangolin (chuan shan jia) The scales of *Manis Penta-dactyla* are the base of a drug that promotes the growth of white blood cells, benefits the circulation, increases milk flow in nursing mothers, reduces swelling, dispels viscous matter from infected wounds, and stimulates the menstrual flow.

Praying mantis (sang piaoi xiao) The eggcase of the murderous female yields a secretion that increases the sperm count while at the same time preventing premature ejaculation. It also stops wetting of the bed.

Rhinoceros (xi jiao) The powdered horn of fabled aphrodisiac property is also useful in reducing fever and maintaining the health. Its use is now limited as however useful for humans, it has had deleterious effects on the Rhinoceros.

Scorpion (xie) The powder obtained by crushing the carapace of the scorpion and the solution achieved by boiling it in water are both effective for the treatment of liver complaints and nervous disorders. They are also worthy antispasmodics, analgesics and effective antidotes.

Spotted deer (lu rong) The horn and velvet antler of *Cervus Nippon* yield one of the most powerful sexual tonics in the Chinese pharmacopoeia. Its most potent essence is obtained by drinking the fresh blood and secretions that ooze from the freshly cut horn.

Tortoise (bie jia) The powdered upper shell clears blockages in the bloodstream and softens tumours. It also reduces fever.

Viper (bai hua she) The much-reduced fluid obtained by boiling the snake's headless body in water is beneficial in treating the aches and pains caused by rheumatism, rids the body of intestinal worms and other parasites and has welcome sedative properties to boot. This fluid is extremely toxic and must be used with caution.

Water buffalo (niu huang) The powdered bezoar (ruminatory hard mass found in the beast's intestines) has the same properties as Rhinoceros Horn, in place of which it is sometimes sold by duplicitous herbalists.

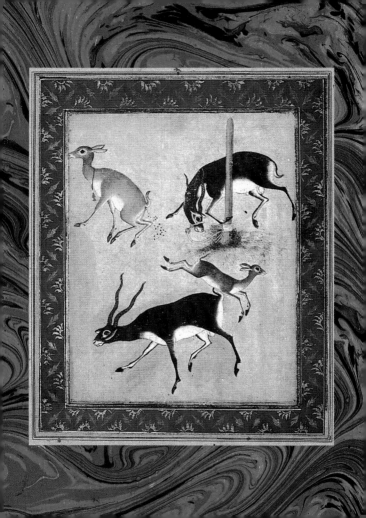

HEALTH AND HOROSCOPE

*Since Man's earliest existence, through succeeding
generations, was there ever a time when the rulers
failed to observe the Sun, Moon and Planets, record
their motions, and expound their meaning? Raise the
head and contemplate the vastness of the Heavens; look
round, and marvel at their manifestations on Earth.
Theirs is the primeval force, and such was related by
the sages of long ago.*

Thus spake Su Ma Ch'ien in the second century BC, by
which time the guiding principles of the Chinese
Horoscope had long been established. Such Horoscopes
differ from those of the **Occident** in many aspects, one
of which is that according to the ways of the **Orient** it is
the year of birth rather than the month that is of **All-
Encompassing Importance**.

The wise men of the east who looked to the heavens for
the paths that preordain our lives, held **Jupiter** in such
high regard that they based their Astrological Timetable
around its path around the sky. The planet takes twelve
years – **The Great Year** – to complete its orbital cycle.
The **Sages** divided the Great Year into **Twelve Earthly
Branches**, each of which corresponds to an ordinary
Occidental year.

In early times, the secrets of things astrological were for the Emperor and his Court alone, but as the Empire expanded, ritual and ceremony came to play a part of increasing importance in Everyday Life and it came to pass that men and women of lesser rank became aware of such matters.

The abstract nature of the Twelve Earthly Branches were beyond the comprehension of many of those of lowly station, and so, one thousand years ago, each of the Branches was assigned the name of an animal and thus that aspect of Chinese Astrology with which those in the West have a nodding acquaintance came into being.

According to the Dictates established a millenium ago, the twelve years are named Rat, Ox, Tiger, Rabbit, Dragon, Snake, Horse, Ram, Monkey, Rooster, Dog and Pig. Those born in a particular year share Certain Common Characteristics, and are prone to illnesses and agues of a Similar Nature.

Those born in the year of the **Rat** are gregarious, intelligent and polite: strong willed, over-critical and petty. And in matters pertaining to health will suffer only minor illnesses during their lives, which can be as short as 65 for those born between three and five of the morning clock to 88 years for those who left the womb between the hours of nine and eleven in the morning.

Determined, conventional and patient: intolerant, prejudiced and headstrong. Such words are oft applied to those born in the year of the **Ox**. Even those who first see the light of day in the two hours prior to eleven o'clock in the morning and who can expect to live well into their eighties, will suffer from many illnesses of a recurring nature, especially those of digestive in origin.

Cautious, optimistic, intelligent – selfish, critical and argumentative **Tigers**, as you stalk your way through life flirting hither and thither as you go, suffer from many minor illnesses, especially colds and influenza brought about by changes in climate.

Oh, youthful, energetic, elegant **Rabbits**, how can you be so obstinate on occasions, so fearful of confrontation and so intolerant of new ideas? Oh lucky Rabbit, as you move through life prospering greatly as you go, your path is unclouded by serious illness.

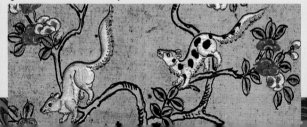

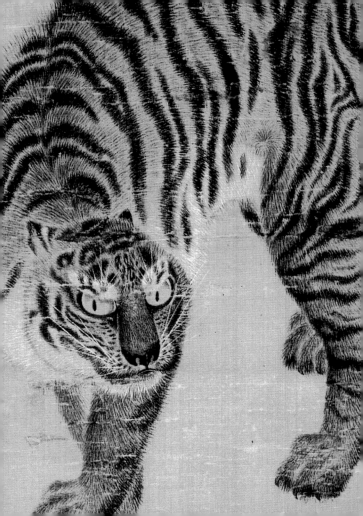

Dragons are strong energetic and authoritative, obstinate, selfish and suspicious of the motives of others. Some Dragons live to Great Age, others burn themselves out long before they have achieved their three score years and ten. The Dragon's health is much affected by the pace they set themselves making them prone to exhaustion, stress and the dreaded Hypertension.

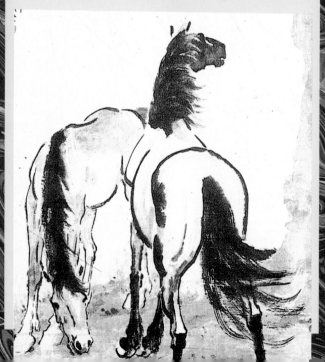

Blessed with wit and dazzlingly attractive to the opposite sex, cursed with black moods and pride, even those **Snakes** who attain Great Age are often plagued by illnesses of a nervous nature.

Active, confident and a natural leader: impatient, hot-tempered and vain. Those born in the year of the **Horse** have the legendary constitution of that most noble beast and can look forward to an illness-free canter through life.

Beware mild, amiable and sensitive **Ram**: take care, you unpunctual, hesitant and obstinate ovine. For although a few of you will reach Great Age, others will arrive at Dame Nature's Abattoir when those born under other signs are in their prime. Refrain from overindulgence in liquids alcoholic, for you are prone to ailments of the liver.

Cunning and wily, wise and warm-hearted, mani-pulative and creative **Monkeys** tend to disregard their health, assuming that their aches and pains are best left to sort themselves out. Sadly, these aches and pains all too often signify something of a Very Serious Nature, too advanced to be treated other than for palliative reasons by the time proper heed of them is taken.

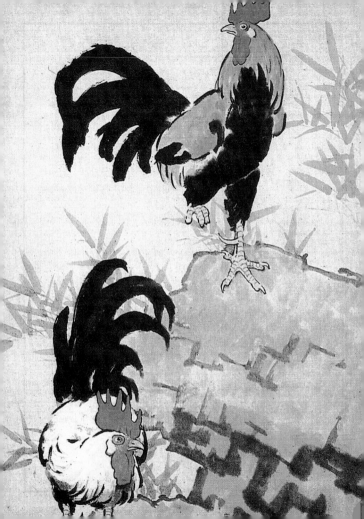

The **Rooster** is king of the barnyard. A bird of great intuitive powers, of scrupulous honesty and high intelligence: a bird that is an impatient exhibitionist and an ill-mannered spendthrift. Many Roosters crow their last while young, others, especially those born in very early or late morning, continue to strut round their domain as they approach their ninetieth year. Roosters catch colds as often as they attempt to catch a glance of themselves in the mirror.

Dogs are active, energetic and clever, if prone to being of a moody, unsettled disposition. They can race towards their ninth, sometimes tenth decade, safe in the knowledge that they are hale of heart and sound of organ, but in their haste, they frequently fall, causing bones to break and blood vessels to burst.

Reserved, hard-working and warm-hearted **Pigs**, well may you be suspicious of the motives of others for which other animal in Astrology is fattened so affectionately only to be led, so innocently, to the slaughter. As you fatten yourself at the trough of life, beware the minor illnesses that others appear to shrug off easily, for if these agues take hold, especially illnesses of a respiratory nature, the outlook may be dark indeed.

DISEASE CURES DISEASE

In the **Eleventh Century** AD a Taoist hermit living in the Chinese province of Sichuan was brought the news that the Prime Minister, one Wang Dan, had sent urgently around the Empire seeking any chemist or physician who had discovered the secret of curing **Smallpox**. His eldest son was dying of the dreaded disease and he was fearful that the rest of his family would succumb.

Answering the summons, the old hermit journeyed to the Imperial Capital bringing with her a number of Smallpox Scabs. She wrapped them in muslin and placed them in the patient's nose. Great was the rejoicing when the youth survived.

This esoteric **Taoist** practice was known then, as now, as **Inoculation**. Though a fable, there is, as ever, a glimmer of truth in it, for the alchemists practised not only in their laboratories, but also experimented on themselves. And thus they discovered that serious diseases could be avoided by introducing a weaker strain of that self-same disease into the body. The Ancient Chinese trusted **Nature**, but it was not until nearly 3000 years later that this effect would be Properly Formulated.

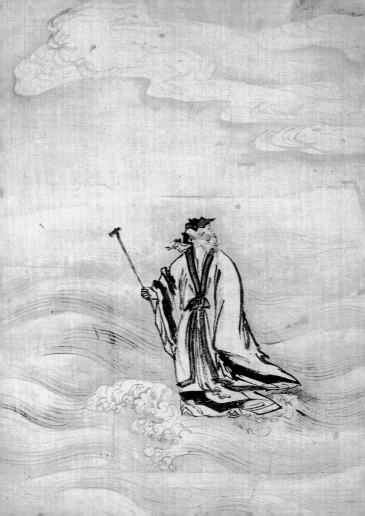

T'AI CHI

Almost one thousand years ago, the venerable **Chang Sang-feng**, a **Taoist** thinker of Some Repute, was musing on the Aggressive Nature of Martial Arts. His dream was to find a way to soften them in form, as a means of developing the spirit.

One day, his attention was caught by a Magpie pecking at a Snake. He noticed how the serpent moved continually and slowly in trying to find a way to outwit its assailant. He became Almost Mesmerized by the yielding quality of the neat, circular movements used by the snake to tease the bird, keeping just out of reach, writhing and curling in graceful motion. Later, he used such movements as the basis of an exercise for the development of self-mastery called *Ch'un* or **Fist**.

Ch'un was adopted by Taoist monks in monasteries and temple schools as a method of integrating the body, mind and spirit by the efficacious combination of movement and spirit. The Holy Men found that in the execution of the **T'ai Chi** (for that is what it came to be called) their minds and bodies became focused. It then gradually metamorphosized into a healing process of a meditative nature in which anyone could participate.

Like most things Chinese, T'ai Chi aims to achieve a balance between peaceful, gentle Yin and active, creative Yang, the imbalances that cause disease being corrected by the mental focusing encouraged by T'ai Chi.

It is Part and Parcel of Chinese Culture, with millions taking part everday in outdoor sessions held in the morning and on the Going Down of the Sun.

The graceful, flowing movements of **T'ai Chi** make it Especially Effective in combating Anxiety and Stress. The exercises improve breathing and posture and are held by Practitioners of the Art to be Islands of Sanity in the Sea of Anxiety.

According to the saintly Chang San-fen, 'the inner strength is rooted in the feet, developed in the thighs, controlled by the waist and expressed through the fingers.'

T'ai Chi uses the image of Water to represent the flow of

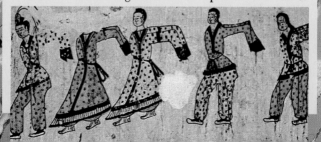

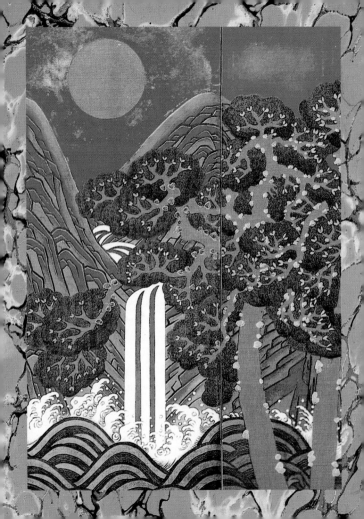

energy, and the symbol of Earth the flow between person and planet. All its movements complement each other: they begin with a stillness and in the words of one expert, 'manifest a sense of revitalization while producing a profound feeling of serenity and well-being.'

The spread of T'ai Chi from Orient to Occident has been Remarkable and those of the West who have become skilled in its Intricacies, maintain that the patience, perseverance, and ability to simplify, adapt and change demanded in its mastery are Worth Much Effort for they hold that of all holistic therapies, T'ai Chi is the most complete, natural and effective.

There are two forms of T'ai Chi, the short, made up of 40 movements each of which flow into each other and the long,which demands completion of upwards of one hundred movements. The former, with no repetitions, takes up to ten minutes to complete; the latter, with repetitions, takes four times that time if the practitioner is to gain maximum benefit.

In the words of one skilled in all aspects of *T'ai Chi*, 'we live in both inner and outer worlds: the inner domain of thought and reflection, the outer of force and action. *T'ai Chi* shows us how to blend these worlds and express a sense of unity and fulfilment.'

THE DOCTOR ASKS; THE PATIENT TELLS

The dictates of our cause in this brief volume precludes the deep Philosophical Dissertation which **Ayurvedic Medicine** so richly deserves. Suffice it to record that in this, the most ancient of medical disciplines, We, and the Universe in which we exist, are controlled by **Five Bhutas** namely **Ether, Fire, Water, Air** and **Earth**. Likewise the Body is made up of **Seven Dhatus** or **Tissues**. Ayurveda strives to ensure that they all **Co-exist** in **Peaceful harmony** thus achieving the physical and mental well-being of all who seek its sanctuary.

It is a widely held belief that Hippocrates is the Father of Occidental Medicine. Those who qualify to practise in its skills Swear an Oath to that most Saintly of Scholars. But we must recognise that he was much influenced by the teachings of Pythagoras who looked to the Teachings of the Indian Mystics for his Inspiration. It is for this reason that much of the nomenclature of Modern Medicine and its Kinsman, Pharmacy, indicate that they are of Indian Origin. A similar study of the Etymology of the Hindi Medical Vocabulary will reveal nothing that is not Hindi in Root and Reason. And thus with Ayurveda, so-called from Ayur meaning *Life* and Veda meaning *Knowledge*.

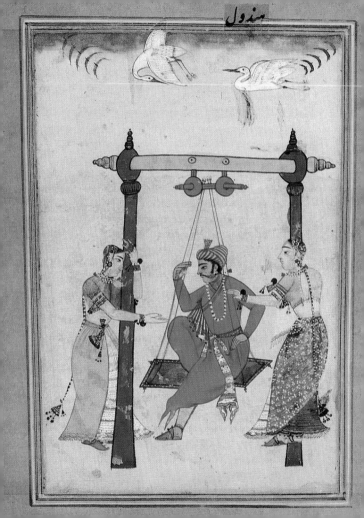

It is known that Principles of Ayurveda were taught around 500 BC at the esteemed University of Benares where that most monumental of Medical Encyclopaedias, the *Samhita*, was written. Much of what is contained in this mightly manuscript has roots that stretch back to the Civilizations that peopled the Nile and Euphrates Valleys as long ago as 3000 BC.

The Ayurveda divides all conditions into four major categories, **Accidental, Physical, Mental** and **Natural**.

Accidental conditions arise from any kind of blow, cut, sting or physical accident and are treated by first aid or, if the accidental condition is of extreme severity, by surgery. Conditions of a Physical Nature include tissue degeneration, inflammations, tumours and blockages, while Mental conditions largely take the form of anger, pride, laziness and fear. And though the pharmacopoeia may be of assistance, the Ayurvedic Practitioner may advise Sympathetic Counselling or Meditation for a patient suffering from such complaints.

Natural conditions are those caused by birth and ageing and may be treated by participating in religious rites and ceremonies.

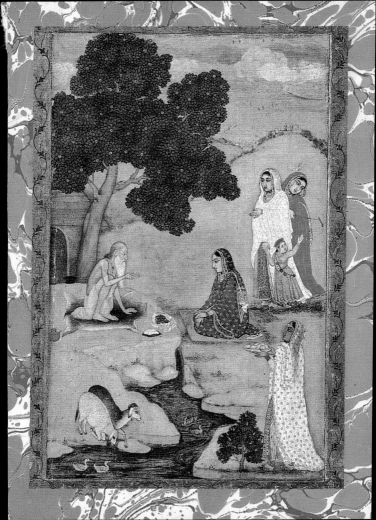

Medicinal treatments involve the use of drugs made from herbs, vegetables and minerals. Attaining the correct balance for a course of drug treatment is a time-consuming process and it can take Many Months of preparation to Achieve the Necessary Balance. Drugs derived from herbs and vegetables are taken when fresh as they lose potency as they age. Conversely, mineral drugs gain in strength the longer they are kept.

Diet is also vital to Ayurvedic Medicine. The physician advises the patient not just what to eat to remedy a particular condition, but also takes account of the weather and season when prescribing a particular dietary regime and tells the patient at what time of day the various foodstuffs on the diet should be eaten. Food must be eaten slowly and chewed well while the patient is in a Beneficial Frame or Mind.

According to the Ayurvedic Principles the **Dhatus** are fed by food in its digested form. Imbalances in the Dietary Intake sicken the Dhatus, leading to Physical and Mental Manifestations. While other matters such as Climate, Physical Surroundings, Sleeping Patterns, Sexual Activities and Age can also affect the Course of a Disease, it is unwise to eat that which makes us ill in the first place.

The Ayurveda categorizes food into six different groups. The first is **The Awed Grains** and includes over twenty varieties of rice, wheat, jowar and the inferior corns usually consumed by the Poor.

Next in importance are the protein-rich **Pods or Legumes** and include the important dhals such as Chana. As a group they tend to produce flatulence and constipation so their intake must be Carefully Controlled.

Oil-yielding Grains make up the third category. They include Sersama, Mustard, Javas and Groundnut. They share a bitter, astringent taste and their use is advocated for external use.

Cooked Foods compose the fourth category. According to the dictates of Ayurvedic Medicine, deer, antelope, cocks, peacocks and sparrows are dry and digestible. Mongoose, hares, camels, tigers, lions, bears, monkeys, cats and jackals are rarely eaten.

Vegetables and **Fruits** such as karavella, which improves the appetite and is useful in the treatment of diabetes and asthma; yam and onions, which are efficaceous in the treatment of piles, and mango which builds tissue; but the king amongst the fruits is the grape (draksha).

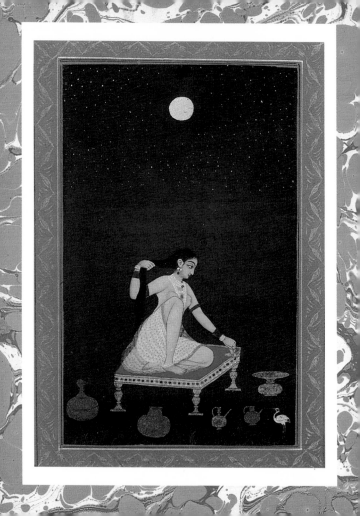

Unlike Occidental Medicine which may be hastily prescribed, the Ayurvedic Practitioner must take time to treat the afflicted as a unique Being, with equally unique balances and imbalances. No Ayurvedic physician would contemplate offering a diagnosis or embark on a course of treatment without first consulting the patients' horoscope, examining waste body fluids, listening to the voice, as well as carrying out a thorough physical examination.

The Doctor asks; the patient tells. The Doctor listens, the patient reflects, The Doctor Counsels; the patient submits, without question and without qualification.

With its roots firmly fixed in the sacred, Ayurveda also involves the repetition of **Mantras**, the participation in Mystic Ceremonies and the practice of **Yoga**. High regard is also given to the use of Refined Oxides and the Power of Precious Stones.

The Ayurvedic Practitioner must be in possession of Diagnostic Skills of almost Psychic Dimensions; and of the Pharmacopoeia, a knowledge deep enough to plumb the accumulated knowledge of time.

Ayurvedic Remedies for all the Family

The following home remedies will prove to be a boon if used in a judicious manner.

Balu-Kadu is a bitter tonic especially suited to children whose dietary intake has become unbalanced, especially if it is Deficient in Carbohydrates. *Arvindasava* is a useful tonic for younger members of the family who will also relish the sweetness of *Wasaka Avaleha* when they are stricken by colds.

The Lady of the House afflicted by Complaints of a Feminine Nature may look to *Ashoka Aristha* for relief and those exhausted by the efforts necessary to bring new life into the world should look to *Balant Kadhu* as a tonic and restorative.

The Master of the House whose sexual prowess has lessened, should partake of either *Sitapalasavan Mishrana* or *Dhatupaustic* pills.

Any member of the family afflicted by summer heat should sip a little sweet, rose flavoured *Gulkand*. Those whose bowels are overloose may well find that *Belphal Moramba* brings calm to the fundamental area of the body.

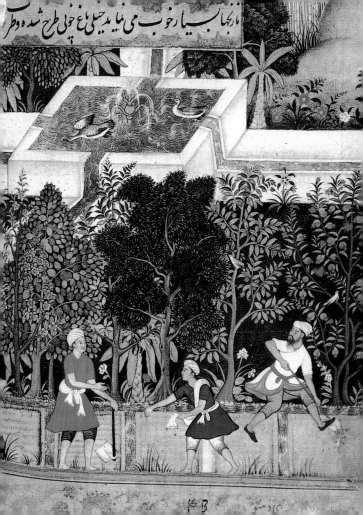

ORIENTAL MEDICINE AND SEX

The mists of time have swirled thicker and thicker since the day when a **Chinese Goat-herd** noticed that the males in his herd were **Especially Active**, attempting practices of a **Sexual Nature** several times in a short space of time.

His curiousity aroused, he kept vigil over a period of weeks,during the course of which he noticed that it was after the herb grazed on a particular patch of weeds that their sexual activities were most marked. And thus, the aphrodisiac properties of *Epigmedium sagittatum*, an aid to male Potency of Particular Power, came to the attention of the Chinese Herbalists who call it *Yin Yang Huo*, which translates roughly as 'horny goat weed'.

Tonics containing this Most Effective herb promote increased secretions of the male hormone and bring about a rise in the production of the male seed. And by expanding the vessels of the Circulatory System, it encourages the flow of hormone-enriched blood to the most sensitive of Body Tissues.

Horn of Rhino and Testes of Tiger

The search for Aphrodisiacs is as old as history, and many and various are the receipts for lotions and potions

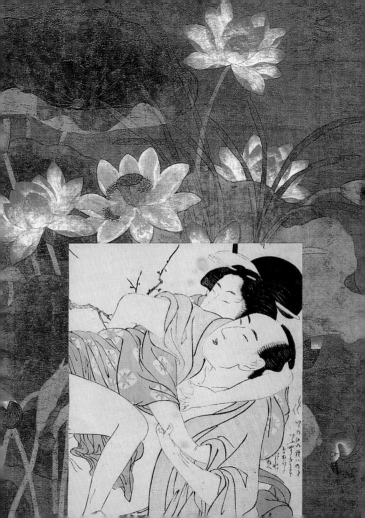

recommended to stimulate the sex drive and lengthen the delights of a Sexual Congress. While those in the Occident place their trust in a dish of oysters or a dash of coriander to heighten the sexual longings those in the Orient have long looked to Horn of Rhinoceros, Testes of Tiger and Penis of Seal to stimulate the Sexual Appetite.

Chinese herbalists have long held that their remedies, as well as promoting long life if used in conjunction with a traditional Chinese diet, also lead to a well-regulated sexual life, and the writings of the sages are Rich in Sexual References.

A man can live a healthy and long life if he carries out an emission frequency of two times monthly or twenty-four times yearly. If at the same time he also pays attention to wholesome food and exercise, he may attain longevity.

Venerable Sun Simiao

This flew in the face of earlier advice;

In Spring, a man can permit himself to ejaculate once in three days. In Summer and Autumn, twice a month. During cold Winter, one should have semen and not ejaculate at all. The way to heaven is to accumulate Yang-essence during Winter. A man will attain longevity if he follows this yardstick. One ejaculation in cold Winter is one hundred times more harmful than in Springtime.

Master Liu Ching

point in the palm of their hand where the tip of a completely flexed index finger touches it and thrice pressing that spot for fifteen seconds.

Sinus and nasal congestion, facial tension and the Miseries of Toothache can all be made to vanish by pressing inwards and upwards on the spaces under cheekbones, directly below the pupils of the eye when staring straight ahead.

And by spreading the right hand, placing the left-hand thumb on the back of the web and the index finger on the corresponding area of the palm and gently massaging for twenty seconds, before repeating the process on the left hand relief is literally on hand for those who have eaten well by not too wisely. This should not, however, be practised by women who are in a delicate condition and refraining from public engagements for the immediate future.

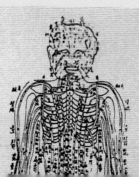

MIND OVER MATTER

There are those who labour under the misapprehension that meditation is a form of self-indulgent and passive introversion practised by those of an eccentric nature. Such misconceptions should be banished from the mind, for meditation is a technique of mind control that has benefits of the most satisfying nature for our health.

Not only does it increase our inner calm and heighten latent powers of creativity, it quickens the decision-making process and Decreases Mental Tension and the negative emotions that can cloud our lives. Meditation at least lessens, at best eliminates stress-related ailments such as migraine and tension headaches, hypertension and, of Especial Interest to the Fair Sex, can deaden the pain too often associated with the monthly flow of blood.

Meditation heightens our powers of awareness and Deep Tranquillity and those who practise it on a regular basis maintain that it represents a journey to the inner self, a journey that is rich in rewards.

Meditation broadens our sense of being and diminishes the personal anxieties and tensions that are the Under-lying Cause of many of the agues to which we are prone.

Meditation which is, in its most basic form, Sitting in Silent Contemplation, is an essential part of Buddhism, Hinduism. Sufism, Christianity and the other Great Religions of the world.

Meditation can be approached in either of two basic ways: Concentration or Detached Focus. Concentration demands that the meditator's attention is focused on a symbol of a meditative nature, be it a sound, a chant or the process of regular breathing. Some find that chanting the Hari Krishna, Aum or other mantra to be a great aid to concentration. As the mind is emptied of the mundane, the thought processes turn inward and as concentration intensifies, the mind transcends thought. The focus of Detached Awareness is 'What is happening now', not to raise conscious thought to a transcendental state but to increase awareness of the present and in so doing gain awareness of the ebb and flow of Human Experience.

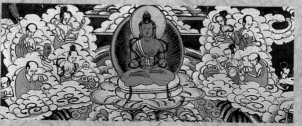

The Buddhist Way

In the fifth century, the Buddhist monk Buddhaghosa described in the *Visuddhimagga* (The Path to Purification) the Buddhist approach to meditation. Its aim is to attain a Unification of Mind by eliminating distraction and to encourage long periods of meditation during which agitation, scepticism and doubt dissolve and are replaced eventually by a feeling of bliss.

As the Seeker of Bliss becomes more and more absorbed in thought an awareness of Infinite Space is acquired, a process known as *Jhana*. But the various levels of *jhana* are of lesser importance than the Ultimate Goal – the Path of Mindfulness which leads, in the end, to Nirvana.

When the meditator comes to perceive every moment of everyday reality as a new event, the ego becomes less and less important, a sense of detachment from worldly experience is achieved, self-interest is abandoned and, in the end, the ego itself ceases to exist.

Meditation can have physical as well as mental benefits. Many of those stricken by asthma have found that the simple breathing techniques practised by those expert in the art of meditation help to control alarming Bronchial Spasms.

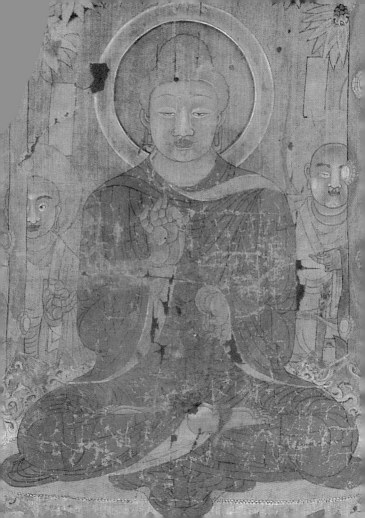

How to Meditate

Refrain from partaking of food or drink for at least half an hour before starting to meditate and find a quiet room where you will not be disturbed. Some practitioners lie down, but many found this Conducive to Sleep rather than an aid to concentration, so many masters of meditation sit upright on a chair, eyes open with hands resting on the lap.

Try to drive thoughts of a troublesome or stimulatory nature from the mind and focus it on one neutral or gently calming thought. Breath in feeling the air entering the nostrils and filling the lungs completely before being expelled slowly. Concentrate on the diaphragm and abdomen, trying to move the former down and making the latter swell. Take as long to empty the lungs as you did to fill them, counting each intake and expulsion of air.

Once the Art of Proper Breathing has been mastered, concentrate on relaxing every area of the body, starting with the head and moving downwards with each breath until your body feels wondrously free of tension.

At first, many thoughts will intrude. Acknowledge them but do not think them through: and once acknowledged sume concentration on the thought of your focus. Many find it a help to focus the thoughts on an object, a favourite photograph, perhaps, or a vase of flowers.

The Meditative State should last for no more than ten minutes and as you become more practised in its art, you will be able to meditate at any time in any place. Many find a few minutes meditation a great help before a meeting in the workplace, especially if the meeting is going to be of a Confrontationary Nature.

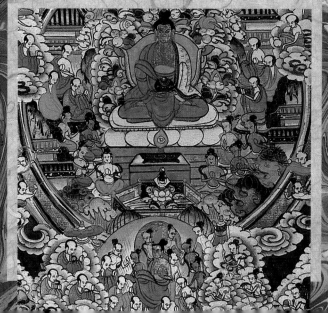

PURE PERFECT POSTURES

The word **Yoga** derives from the Sanskrit *yuj* which means 'to bind together', and it is through Yoga that Man seeks how to **Find Union** with the **State of Being**.

Stone Seals uncovered in the age-old city of Mohenjo-Daro in Present-day Pakistan depict men sitting in cross-legged positions that are familiar today to those versed in the skills of yoga. These seals have existed for four thousand years, but for most of that time Deep Knowledge of yoga was restricted to an elite band of philosophers and meditators, the Gurus, who chose the hermit's existence, passing on their knowledge to a Small Band of followers, so ensuring its exclusivity.

It is only in this, the Twentieth of Occidental Centuries, that Yoga has been made accessible to Common Folk. In India, in such high regard is it held, that the Relevant Authorities encourage the teaching of physical yoga exercises to all schoolchildren.

You must have Complete Trust in your Chosen Teacher, and to achieve the State of Mind sought after the advice must be Devotedly followed. Only so can the Art of Concentration be mastered, essential from the further mastery of the postures known to Yogis as Asanas.

Sidhasana is the posture for Meditation, sitting cross-legged in the way of on old-fashioned tailor.

Padmasana the Lotus Seat, so-called after the lotus floating perfectly over the waters, sets the mind free to soar over the temptation of the flesh; and nervous system is marvellously calmed.

During **Yoga-Mudra**, breathe deeply in and deeply out. Bend forward to bring the forehead into contact with the floor in order to restore the organs of the abdominal cavity.

When in the most beneficial posture of **Supta-Vajrasana** our conscious thoughts are guided to the solar plexus and the region of the heart. In so doing, the nervous system is affected in a stimulatory Way and the Glandular Functions invigorated.

Ardha-Matsyendrasana is a difficult posture that takes much practice, but when adopting this Asana backbones are strengthened benefitting the nervous system, the liver, pancreas, spleen and intestines.

In **Salabhasana** lying on the stomach and raising legs in the grasshopper style (that gives this asana its name) is efficaceous in achieving cures for complaints of constipatory nature.

To accomplish **Dhanurasana,** lie on the floor, face down. Inhale slowly and reach back to grasp both ankles, arch the back and retain this position for as long as possible. Doing so stimulates glandular activity with fruitful results for those of both sexes unable to match expectation and performance in the bed chamber.

Mayura equivalents itself with the peacock, and this posture reminds us of the way in which that most beautiful of avians spreads its tail. Achieving the necessary balance takes much practice. It cleanses the digestive organs, and its therapeutic effect on the pancreas gland makes it a valuable ally in the prevention and cure of diabetes.

Normal vision is preserved and concentration improved by the **Bru-Madya-Drishti** asana. Adopt the Padmasana position and then inhale deeply before breathing regularly and concentrating on a spot between the eyebrows, above the bridge of the nose. Maintain this until fatigue is felt, relax for a moment and then repeat the exercise, this time looking at the tip of the nose – again until fatigue is experienced.

This entire volume could have been taken up with a discussion of how to achieve **Sarvagansana**, the most important posture for beneficial effect. Suffice it to say that it such a boon to the entire organism that it should be practised several times each day. Those who have mastered its intricacies claim that no medicine can match the feeling of well-being achieved in but two months.

Breathing correctly whilst in the **Viparati-Karani** posture is excellent for those who experience breathing difficulties and those with colds or tonsilitis. It is of especial importance to women who wish to retain a youthful appearance for the flow of blood to the skin and muscles of the face and tones the facial muscles.

Sirshasana, the Yoga head stand, is the third in importance in the hierarchy of the Asanas. It nourishes the brain, heightening powers of concentration and speeding up thought processes. It eases the strain on the heart. It improves vision and encourages deep sleep. Sadly, those with high blood pressure must refrain from its regular practice.

Assuming **Matsyasana** directs the mind towards the thyroid and, as the chest is arched forward and the top of the head touches the floor, stiff necks are eased as are colds and troublesome tonsils.

Breathe in while lying on the back during **Paschi-motana**. Completing the position under the guidance of the Guru strengthens the nerves and improves the condition of the sexual organs, whilst keeping diabetic tendencies at bay.

Nauli, the most difficult of asanas, is well worth mastering for its regenerative effect on the deep-seated muscles of the back and its soothing effect on the organs of the abdomen. It is especial importance for those who wish to lead a life of continence, preventing as it does, nocturnal emissions of a semenal nature.

Bhujangasana, the Cobra posture, involves moving the body into a snake-like position, thus regenerating the kidneys and stimulating the thyroid to such an extent that those suffering from excessive growth of this gland must refrain from this exercise.

Kneeling in the **Ardha-Bhujangasana** posture, elasticity of the hip is encouraged and fatty deposits in that region are discouraged.

Savasana, the corpse posture, should be performed after the sequence of Asanas taught by the Teacher have been achieved. It relaxes the body. Lying on the back, arms close to the body and extended as far as possible, feet and legs similarly stretched, breathing is slowed down. The muscles relax, beginning with the feet, moving upwards. Blood pressure is reduced and Peace Reigns. Ten minutes of this Asana is more beneficial than eight hours in the Arms of Morpheus.

Each Teacher or Guru develops a particular Way of Teaching; an individual Way to help a willing pupil achieve Perfection of Mind and Body.

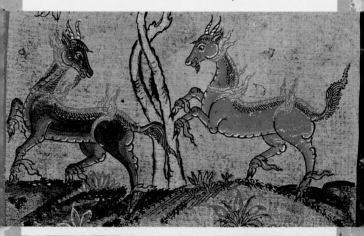

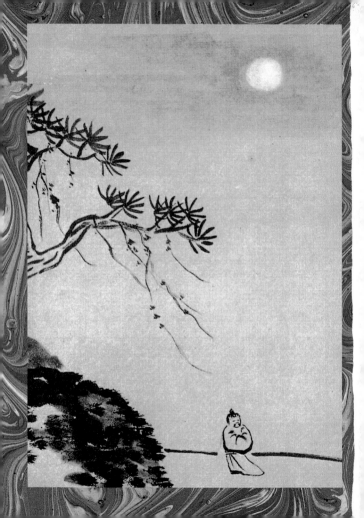

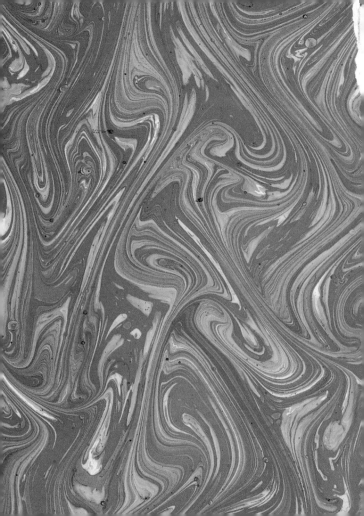